HELLO!

Kate here. Thank you for choosing the How To Be Unbreakable Field Journal to support you on your journey to becoming Unbreakable!

I made this journal to help you put into practice what you learned in my book, "Becoming Unbreakable: How To Build A Body You Love To Live In". *(You don't have to have read the book to use this journal, but it sure does help!)*

The world is awash in the myths that you can reach "too late" while you're still alive, and that body care is simply "too complicated" to figure out. Both of these sentiments are utter nonsense. And you're going to prove it as the caretaker of your body.

I wanted to give you a heads-up about the resources that are available to you as embark on this journey...

First, this journal. Keep it somewhere you'll be able to find it easily. That makes it easier to pull it out and track the data you've gathered from your experiments. You'll find duplicates of several pages in this journal so that you can track your journey over time.

Second, the "Becoming Unbreakable" book comes with a bonus to take you further into the concepts in the book itself. You can find that at www.theunbreakablebody.com/book-bonus.

Finally, my Unbreakable Body workout program has helped over a thousand folks to build their body with safe and effective physical training. I'd love for you to take the program, too. You can learn more about it at www.theunbreakablebody.com.

Wishing you the best on your journey,

Kate

BECOMING UNBREAKABLE

is an adventure that will take you more places than you could have dreamed, and that will teach you more about yourself than you ever imagined.

Welcome to the journey of a lifetime.

It is never "too late".

It is never "too complicated" for you.

THIS IS THE FIELD JOURNAL OF

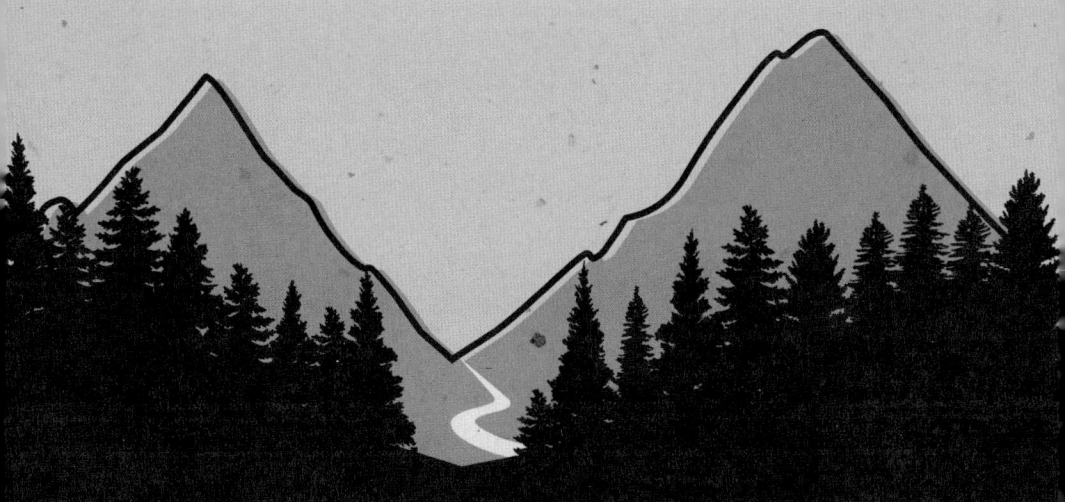

CULTIVATE YOUR UNBREAKABLE VISION

> How do you want to feel?
> What do you want to be able to do?

> How resilient and resistant to do you want to be to aches and pains?

> What does it look like to live your life as an Unbreakable human?

These are just a few of the questions you can reflect on as you begin drafting your vision of what becoming UNBREAKABLE means to you.

As you fill in the next page with your unique vision, decide that whatever your mind and spirit can dream up, you're capable of achieving it. You may not know how yet, but nothing's "too complicated" for you, remember?

You don't have to get it "perfect" the first time through. For one thing, "perfect" doesn't exist. On top of that, your vision is going to go through adaptations and adjustments as time goes on.

Becoming UNBREAKABLE is a life-long journey, and the journey itself is as much a part of the vision as the goals you're hoping to achieve.

Come back to your vision every now and again and update it so it still aligns with who you are and where you're heading.

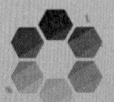

MY UNBREAKABLE VISION

To me, becoming Unbreakable looks like...

To me, becoming Unbreakable feels like...

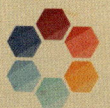

EXPLORING YOUR BODY ECOSYSTEM

Now that you've crafted your Unbreakable vision, it's time to set off on the journey to becoming Unbreakable. The first thing to do is to start seeing your body as an ecosystem and yourself as its caretaker. From there, you can figure out what's here, what's not, and how to make life here, in your body, as hospitable as possible.

In nature, ecosystem are dynamic entities that are always in flux. They are actually always responding and adapting accordingly to the ever-shifting environment. They are influenced by both internal and external factors. What flourishes in an ecosystem is a result of how that ecosystem is managed, worked with, and supported. The same is true for your body.

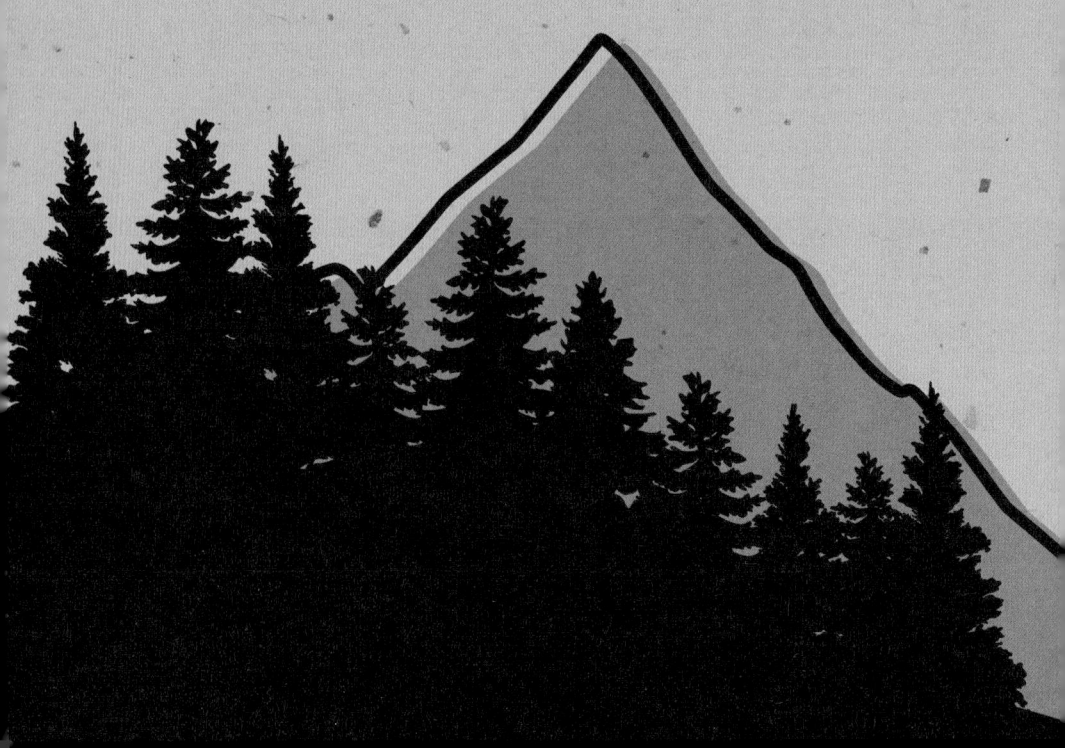

On the next page, write or draw what your body ecosystem is like today. And remember, while you will likely start with the physical elements of your body ecosystem, your ecosystem doesn't end there.

Consider your daily life, your work, any stressors you're dealing with, your emotions or worries, and any other aspects of your inner and outer environments in which your body ecosystem lives.

PS: I've included four body ecosystem pages so that you can fill out a new one each quarter over the course of a year. Your body ecosystem is bound to change over time, so set a reminder and do a new exploration every three months!

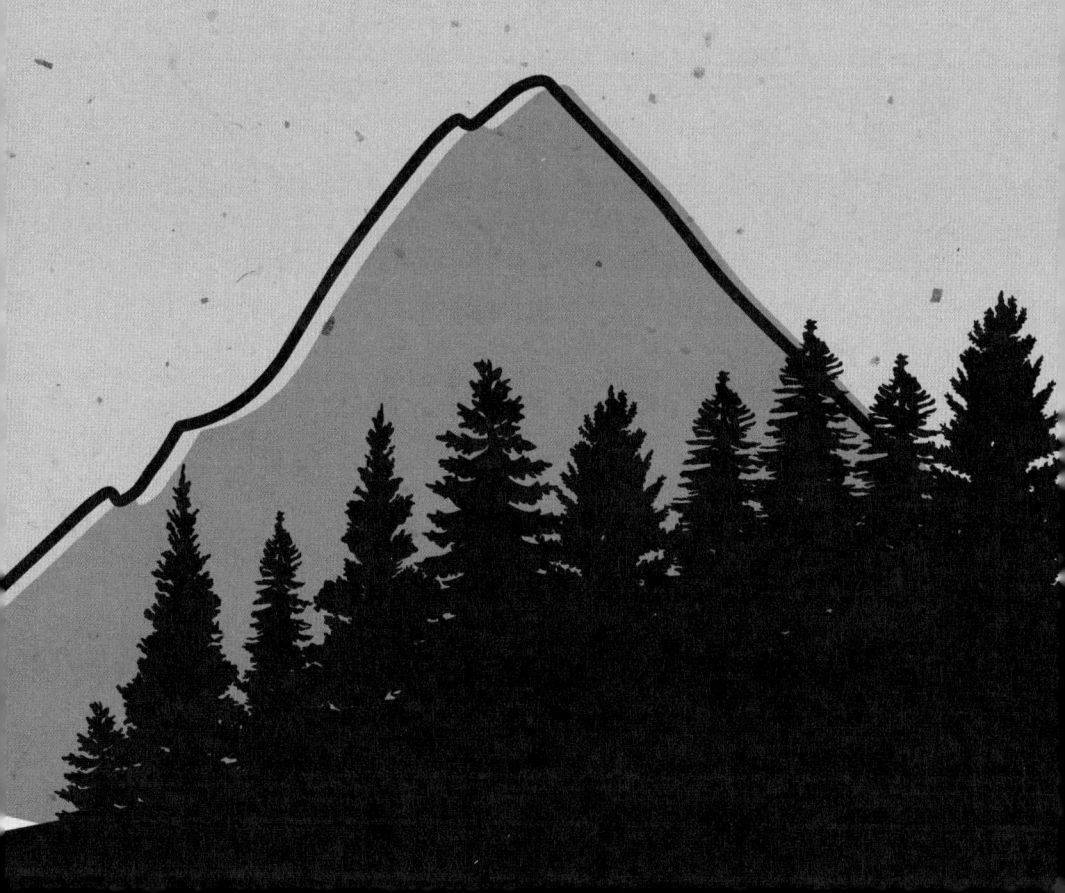

YOUR BODY IS AN ECOSYSTEM.
AND YOU ARE ITS CARETAKER.

Write or draw what your body ecosystem is like today.

What is here? What's not here that you wish it was? What does your body ecosystem need to make life here as hospitable as possible for you? How resistant do you feel? How resilient do you feel?

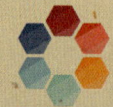

Date:

YOUR BODY IS AN ECOSYSTEM. AND YOU ARE ITS CARETAKER.

Write or draw what your body ecosystem is like today.

What is here? What's not here that you wish it was? What does your body ecosystem need to make life here as hospitable as possible for you? How resistant do you feel? How resilient do you feel?

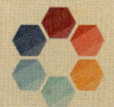

Date:

YOUR BODY IS AN ECOSYSTEM.
AND YOU ARE ITS CARETAKER.

Write or draw what your body ecosystem is like today.

What is here? What's not here that you wish it was? What does your body ecosystem need to make life here as hospitable as possible for you? How resistant do you feel? How resilient do you feel?

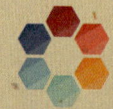

Date:

YOUR BODY IS AN ECOSYSTEM.
AND YOU ARE ITS CARETAKER.

Write or draw what your body ecosystem is like today.

What is here? What's not here that you wish it was? What does your body ecosystem need to make life here as hospitable as possible for you? How resistant do you feel? How resilient do you feel?

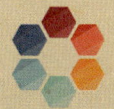

Date:

SIX PILLARS SELF ASSESSMENT

The Six Pillars are an easy-to-follow framework for building your body to have a strong base of fitness. Reflect on your Six Pillars and use the figure on the next page to fill in your self-assessment of each of the Pillars. Here are questions to ask yourself to aid you in your assessment:

Mobile Shoulders

Are your shoulders stiff and tight feeling? Do you feel like your neck and upper shoulders get really tight and tender? Have you had past shoulder aches or injuries?

Mobile Hips

Are your hips stiff and tight, or do you feel "click-y" or when you move them? Do your hips limit your movement? Have you had past aches or injuries to your hip area?

Fill this information into the figure in a manner that suits you best... You could write it out, use a numbering system, or use drawings to express your self-assessment.

Note: I've given you four self-assessment pages so that you can do a new assessment every quarter over the course of a year.

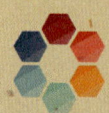

Strong Posture

Do you feel like your posture isn't as stacked as it could be? Do you get aches or stiffness in your back or neck? Do you feel like you can be comfortable in any position, whether sitting, standing, or moving about?

Strong Torso

Does your breathing feel as deep, full, and restorative as it could be? Do you feel like you can adequately brace your body to pick things up, bend over, or move about without worrying that you'll strain or tweak a muscle?

Strong Glutes

Are you doing any sort of resistance training that targets your glutes? Have your glutes felt achy or stiff lately?

Strong Feet

Do your feet feel good most of the time? Have you had issues with plantar fasciitis, ankle sprains, bunions, or other foot/lower leg issues?

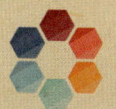

SIX PILLARS SELF ASSESSMENT

Strong Posture

Mobile Shoulders

Strong Torso

Mobile Hips

Strong Glutes

Strong Feet

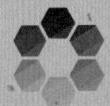

Date:

SIX PILLARS SELF ASSESSMENT

Strong Posture

Mobile Shoulders

Strong Torso

Mobile Hips

Strong Glutes

Strong Feet

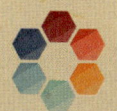

Date:

SIX PILLARS SELF ASSESSMENT

Strong Posture

Mobile Shoulders

Strong Torso

Mobile Hips

Strong Glutes

Strong Feet

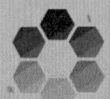

Date:

SIX PILLARS SELF ASSESSMENT

Strong Posture

Mobile Shoulders

Strong Torso

Mobile Hips

Strong Glutes

Strong Feet

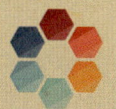

Date:

EXPLORER'S MINDSET PROCESS

Explore

- ✓ Collect data in your body ecosystem
- ✓ Take note of any stories or emotions that are tethered to your data
- ✓ Remember to use curious compassion as you explore

Experiment

- ✓ Select the response you'd like to experiment on and use the Three What's & A Who Question Framework to determine an experiment you can do to influence that response (Remember that you can experiment on stories and emotions as well!)
- ✓ Set the parameters for your experiment
- ✓ Do your experiment

Curate

- ✓ Track the results of your experiments
- ✓ Make note of the things that worked the way you'd hoped and use them to make a truly tailored protocol for what makes you Unbreakable

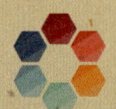

PUTTING YOUR EXPLORER'S MINDSET TO WORK

Finally, the moment you've either been excitedly waiting for, or you've been dreading... Doing experiments to find what signals get your body to respond in a way you really love.

You might be excited to start experimenting because you're ready to start feeling better. And, you might be full of dread right now because you're not sure where to start, or you've tried things in the past and they didn't seem to work.

If you feel either or both of these, congratulations! You're a typical human being!

Here are few tips if you're unsure where to start:

> Remember that it's often a web of signals that contribute to how your body responds. You can experiment with exercise and the various styles of it that are out there to see how your body responds to them.

> But also, consider that your lifestyle, how you listen to your body, what kind of media and information you consume, and past experiences you've had living in your body, are valuable realms that may contain worthy experiments that could help your body respond favorably, too.

> And if you're still in need of some ideas, head on over to the Becoming Unbreakable book bonus page where you can find more inspiration for your experiments. www.theunbreakablebody.com/book-bonus

PS: I've given you enough pages to do 15 experiments. That might take you the whole year to do that many experiments, or you might do that many in the first three months. It's your journal, use these pages as frequently as you see fit.

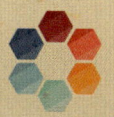

Experiment:

Date started:

What external signals may have contributed to this response?

What internal signals may have contributed to this response?

What's the opportunity here?

Who can help?

What's your hypothesis?

What are the parameters you'll set for this experiment?

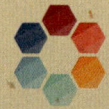

Experiment:

Date started:

Keep any notes and interesting tidbits that you think are worth tracking while doing this experiment here:

What was the outcome/what did you learn?

If the outcome was something worth curating into your regular routine, or as something you should do again should you face this situation in the future, be sure to track it in your Curated Protocols list at the end of this section.

Date:

Experiment:

Date started:

What external signals may have contributed to this response?

What internal signals may have contributed to this response?

What's the opportunity here?

Who can help?

What's your hypothesis?

What are the parameters you'll set for this experiment?

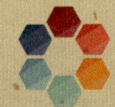

Experiment:

Date started:

Keep any notes and interesting tidbits that you think are worth tracking while doing this experiment here:

What was the outcome/what did you learn?

If the outcome was something worth curating into your regular routine, or as something you should do again should you face this situation in the future, be sure to track it in your Curated Protocols list at the end of this section.

Date:

Experiment:

Date started:

What external signals may have contributed to this response?

What internal signals may have contributed to this response?

What's the opportunity here?

Who can help?

What's your hypothesis?

What are the parameters you'll set for this experiment?

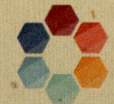

Experiment:

Date started:

Keep any notes and interesting tidbits that you think are worth tracking while doing this experiment here:

What was the outcome/what did you learn?

If the outcome was something worth curating into your regular routine, or as something you should do again should you face this situation in the future, be sure to track it in your Curated Protocols list at the end of this section.

Date:

Experiment:

Date started:

What external signals may have contributed to this response?

What internal signals may have contributed to this response?

What's the opportunity here?

Who can help?

What's your hypothesis?

What are the parameters you'll set for this experiment?

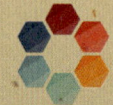

Experiment:

Date started:

Keep any notes and interesting tidbits that you think are worth tracking while doing this experiment here:

What was the outcome/what did you learn?

If the outcome was something worth curating into your regular routine, or as something you should do again should you face this situation in the future, be sure to track it in your Curated Protocols list at the end of this section.

Date:

Experiment:

Date started:

What external signals may have contributed to this response?

What internal signals may have contributed to this response?

What's the opportunity here?

Who can help?

What's your hypothesis?

What are the parameters you'll set for this experiment?

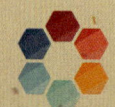

Experiment:

Date started:

Keep any notes and interesting tidbits that you think are worth tracking while doing this experiment here:

What was the outcome/what did you learn?

If the outcome was something worth curating into your regular routine, or as something you should do again should you face this situation in the future, be sure to track it in your Curated Protocols list at the end of this section.

Date:

Experiment:

Date started:

What external signals may have contributed to this response?

What internal signals may have contributed to this response?

What's the opportunity here?

Who can help?

What's your hypothesis?

What are the parameters you'll set for this experiment?

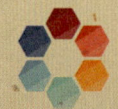

Experiment:

Date started:

Keep any notes and interesting tidbits that you think are worth tracking while doing this experiment here:

What was the outcome/what did you learn?

If the outcome was something worth curating into your regular routine, or as something you should do again should you face this situation in the future, be sure to track it in your Curated Protocols list at the end of this section.

Date:

Experiment:

Date started:

What external signals may have contributed to this response?

What internal signals may have contributed to this response?

What's the opportunity here?

Who can help?

What's your hypothesis?

What are the parameters you'll set for this experiment?

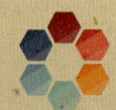

Experiment:

Date started:

Keep any notes and interesting tidbits that you think are worth tracking while doing this experiment here:

What was the outcome/what did you learn?

If the outcome was something worth curating into your regular routine, or as something you should do again should you face this situation in the future, be sure to track it in your Curated Protocols list at the end of this section.

Date:

Experiment:

Date started:

What external signals may have contributed to this response?

What internal signals may have contributed to this response?

What's the opportunity here?

Who can help?

What's your hypothesis?

What are the parameters you'll set for this experiment?

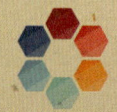

Experiment:

Date started:

Keep any notes and interesting tidbits that you think are worth tracking while doing this experiment here:

What was the outcome/what did you learn?

If the outcome was something worth curating into your regular routine, or as something you should do again should you face this situation in the future, be sure to track it in your Curated Protocols list at the end of this section.

Date:

Experiment:

Date started:

What external signals may have contributed to this response?

What internal signals may have contributed to this response?

What's the opportunity here?

Who can help?

What's your hypothesis?

What are the parameters you'll set for this experiment?

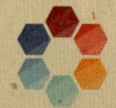

Experiment:

Date started:

Keep any notes and interesting tidbits that you think are worth tracking while doing this experiment here:

What was the outcome/what did you learn?

If the outcome was something worth curating into your regular routine, or as something you should do again should you face this situation in the future, be sure to track it in your Curated Protocols list at the end of this section.

Date:

Experiment:

Date started:

What external signals may have contributed to this response?

What internal signals may have contributed to this response?

What's the opportunity here?

Who can help?

What's your hypothesis?

What are the parameters you'll set for this experiment?

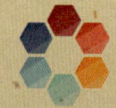

Experiment:

Date started:

Keep any notes and interesting tidbits that you think are worth tracking while doing this experiment here:

What was the outcome/what did you learn?

If the outcome was something worth curating into your regular routine, or as something you should do again should you face this situation in the future, be sure to track it in your Curated Protocols list at the end of this section.

Date:

Experiment:

Date started:

What external signals may have contributed to this response?

What internal signals may have contributed to this response?

What's the opportunity here?

Who can help?

What's your hypothesis?

What are the parameters you'll set for this experiment?

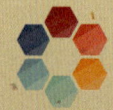

Experiment:

Date started:

Keep any notes and interesting tidbits that you think are worth tracking while doing this experiment here:

What was the outcome/what did you learn?

If the outcome was something worth curating into your regular routine, or as something you should do again should you face this situation in the future, be sure to track it in your Curated Protocols list at the end of this section.

Date:

Experiment:

Date started:

What external signals may have contributed to this response?

What internal signals may have contributed to this response?

What's the opportunity here?

Who can help?

What's your hypothesis?

What are the parameters you'll set for this experiment?

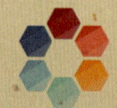

Experiment:

Date started:

Keep any notes and interesting tidbits that you think are worth tracking while doing this experiment here:

What was the outcome/what did you learn?

If the outcome was something worth curating into your regular routine, or as something you should do again should you face this situation in the future, be sure to track it in your Curated Protocols list at the end of this section.

Date:

Experiment:

Date started:

What external signals may have contributed to this response?

What internal signals may have contributed to this response?

What's the opportunity here?

Who can help?

What's your hypothesis?

What are the parameters you'll set for this experiment?

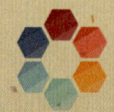

Experiment:

Date started:

Keep any notes and interesting tidbits that you think are worth tracking while doing this experiment here:

What was the outcome/what did you learn?

If the outcome was something worth curating into your regular routine, or as something you should do again should you face this situation in the future, be sure to track it in your Curated Protocols list at the end of this section.

Date:

Experiment:

Date started:

What external signals may have contributed to this response?

What internal signals may have contributed to this response?

What's the opportunity here?

Who can help?

What's your hypothesis?

What are the parameters you'll set for this experiment?

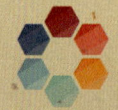

Experiment:

Date started:

Keep any notes and interesting tidbits that you think are worth tracking while doing this experiment here:

What was the outcome/what did you learn?

If the outcome was something worth curating into your regular routine, or as something you should do again should you face this situation in the future, be sure to track it in your Curated Protocols list at the end of this section.

Date:

Experiment:

Date started:

What external signals may have contributed to this response?

What internal signals may have contributed to this response?

What's the opportunity here?

Who can help?

What's your hypothesis?

What are the parameters you'll set for this experiment?

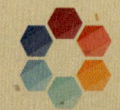

Experiment:

Date started:

Keep any notes and interesting tidbits that you think are worth tracking while doing this experiment here:

What was the outcome/what did you learn?

If the outcome was something worth curating into your regular routine, or as something you should do again should you face this situation in the future, be sure to track it in your Curated Protocols list at the end of this section.

Date:

MY CURATED LIST OF SIGNALS & PROTOCOLS THAT MAKE ME UNBREAKABLE

Use these pages to note both the singular signals that give you a response you prefer, and to keep track of a specific series of signals that help you through body responses you don't prefer, such as "My Low Back Pain Protocol".

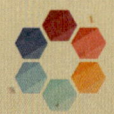

MY CURATED LIST OF SIGNALS & PROTOCOLS THAT MAKE ME UNBREAKABLE

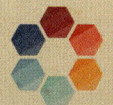

MY CURATED LIST OF SIGNALS & PROTOCOLS THAT MAKE ME UNBREAKABLE

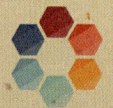

Made in the USA
Middletown, DE
21 January 2022